Anxiety In Relationships Guidebook

The Ultimate Guide To Stop Negative Thinking, Jealousy And Panic Attacks, Understand Attachment And Fear Of Abandonment To Overcome Couple Conflicts

John Myers

&

Ashley Anita Gray

TABLE OF CONTENTS

INTRODUCTION

Thank you very much for purchasing this book. To you, the idea of being in a relationship where you take care of everything and everyone and continually blame yourself for the consequences of others may seem normal. It may not seem unreasonable that you put your needs aside to give the other person exactly what they want as you walk away without once again. You may not know that you are being exploited or that there is a way to stop being exploited by the other person. At this point, you may have no idea that these same behaviors are what contribute to the dysfunction experienced in your relationships.From this experience you will emerge a stronger and more self-confident person, a person who can immediately recognize a good relationship from a bad one. is able to cultivate the lasting love you crave.
Enjoy.

CHAPTER 1 - Secrets You Must Never Keep

SECRETS

There is no standard way of handling a relationship. And this isbecause people are different. The things that excite one personmight not be remotely close to what excites another person.

Also, some people are comfortable with letting out all their secrets totheir partners, whereas some people feel that they should keep some secrets to themselves.

By all means, there's nothing wrong with keeping a secret, but you had better first weigh its impact once it comes to light. The followingare examples of secrets that would not be okay to withhold from yourpartner.

Debt

In these harsh economic times, you might have been forced to approach a financial institution and asked for a loan or loans. There's nothing wrong with taking a loan because, at the end of the day, it is a move calculated to help you. But then you have to disclose to your partner that you are servicing debt, especially if it is a big amount, and you are struggling with it. By failing to disclose to your partner early on and waiting until you default on payments and start to play cat and mouse games with your bank, you put your partner through shame and give them a reason to believe you are crooked.

Playing Their Part Well

In a relationship, both partners should play certain roles so that their relationship might become strong. In some relationships, there's a tremendous power imbalance, to the point that one partner practically slaves for the other.

If you feel that your partner is not pulling their weight, do not make the mistake of keeping it a secret. By making it seem okay that they are not acting, completing the responsibilities they should, you only encourage them to become worse. Asking your spouse to perform their duties will not result in them running away, but rather, it will cause them to respect you more because you have a stand.

History of Drug Abuse

You might think that all your drug-fueled escapades as a young adultshould stay in the past, and to an extent, it is okay. But your partner deserves to know what kind of terrible life-altering experiences you have gone through. Mostly, drug abuse is just a symptom of a deep- seated issue; the drugs offer you an escape window into an alternate world where that problem exists no more. By opening up to your partner about your drug problem, they will help you address any negative changes you might have developed as a result of your dependence on drugs. You may have stopped taking heavy drugs, butare you totally drug-free, or you keep taking some on the low? You should also let your partner know if you still take drugs in secret.

Inability to Have Kids

In the days of long ago, when a man and a woman got together intending to start a family, and then they were unable to get a baby, itwas usually blamed on the woman. But advancement in science has shown us that even a man can be the cause of not getting a baby. Mostof us know whether or not we are injured in that area. So, it is important to disclose to your partner that you do not have the ability to participate in bringing a child to this planet. You should not worry about whether they will want to leave you after finding out this, but you should just be frank with them.

Being Depressed

Do not act as if you possess superhuman strength. You are only mortal. From time to time, you will come down with depression. The symptoms of depression are numerous, but even then, some people are really good at masking these symptoms. Do not be one of them.

The real reason why you have a partner and not living a single life is so that you may have a helper in the season of pain. It is unfortunate that you are depressed already, but do not make it worse by hiding it from your partner. Your partner will appreciate it if you are honest about what you are going through.

Poor Sexual Intimacy

One of the things that bring partners close together is quality sex. A relationship devoid of quality sex usually creates room for resentment. Before long, the former lovers turn into passive-aggressive enemies, and in the worst-case scenario, they part their ways. Different people have different ideas of what constitutes great sex, but if it seems to you that your partner has a poor game in bed, bring it to light. It is nothing to be ashamed of. But then you want to express your point without making fun of your partner or making them feel disrespected. For both of you to be sexually satisfied, you should both do what the other one likes.

A Kid Somewhere

Maybe in your late teens, you went out with a certain person and had sex that resulted in the conception of an unplanned baby. When the baby was given birth to, it was sent to your grandparents or even put up for adoption. Now you have met someone that you fancy and want to start a family with them. Should you disclose to them that you have a baby somewhere? Yes! It is called being honest about your past, and your partner will appreciate it. There are some things we did in the past that have no potential of coming up in our future as long as they were resolved, but then there are some things that we did in the past that always have a probability of affecting our future, and your unplanned kid is one of them.

Medical Health Issues

When two people form a relationship together, they are about sharing their lives. What if one of them could have a virus infection? They would pass it on to their partner. Ensure that you disclose to your partner any health issue you might have, especially if it is a big health problem like cancer or HIV. Will they want to leave you after hearing about your medical condition? Probably! But then think of it this way; you want to be in a relationship with someone that accepts you fully, and when someone runs away from you, that's no loss, but rather an opportunity to meet someone that adores you.

Your True Personality

For some reason, the media teaches us that we should all aspire to be extroverts so that the world may love us. But that's a big depart from reality. There's a big population of people out there who are not comfortable with being the center of attention. They are known as introverts. If you are one of them, do not pretend to be an extrovert so that your partner may like you more, but rather put it in the open that you are an introvert, and that from time to time, you will require to withdraw from your partner so that you may refill your emotional and mental resources.

The Foods You Like

Apart from sex, nothing brings couples together, like good food. But then again, it is a question of preferences. Do not assume that just because you like a certain food that your partner must like it too. Our tastes are different, and they are influenced by a variety of things, including our culture, background, social class, and education. Disclose to your partner the foods that you like indulging in and not suffer silently by forcing yourself to consume what your partner likes even though you do not. Such scenarios normally play out when the partners come from different cultures.

CHAPTER 2 - Types of Codependent Behavior

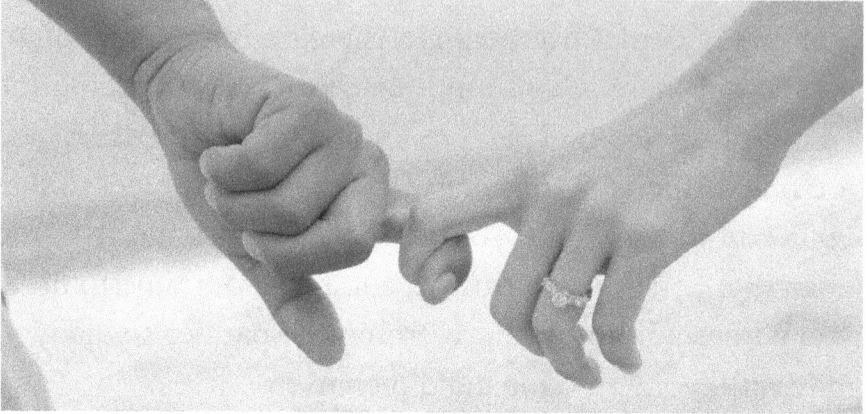

One of the biggest problems with codependent behavior is the fact that many people do not recognize the various forms that it can take just because the term "codependent" is a
single term that doesn't mean that it only has one face. Instead, it's a bit like ice cream. Even though ice cream is one type of food, it comes in many, many flavors. The very same thing can be said about codependency. Despite it being one condition, it can come in many, many forms. Therefore, you must learn the different faces of codependent behavior to recognize the signs that you are in a codependent relationship.

Abusive Behavior

The most extreme type of codependent behavior is abusive behavior. This is the category most people are already familiar with, and so it isthe one that they readily associate with codependent relationships. Ofthe different types of abuses, physical abuse is one of the most extreme, and fortunately, one of the least common. More often than not, the types of relationships affected by physical abuse are parent/child relationships and husband/wife relationships. It is rare that any type of friendship suffers physical abuse, especially to the degree of what is needed to constitute a codependent relationship.

In the case of the parent/child relationship, physical abuse often comes in the form of punishment. A parent will hit their child as a form of reprimand for an act that is considered wrong and undesirable. Many people have physically punished their children from time to time, especially when they do something dangerous that causes their parents to react emotionally. However, slapping a child's hand or even giving them a whack on the backside does not constitute physical abuse as such. Instead, physical abuse is when the parent beats their child relentlessly.

Furthermore, implements such as leather belts, wooden spoons, or thelike also point to abuse. You do not need to use a belt to get the pointacross; therefore, such an act is extreme, indicating a deeper, more sinister root cause. Beating a child is often done to gain control over their behavior, which is where the codependent nature of the act comes into play. Any time a person tries to control the thoughts, feelings, or actions of another person, they are engaging in codependent behavior.

Finally, there is a form of abuse that is psychological. This is the most elaborate form as it requires a great deal of thought and planning to pull off. Therefore, even though psychological abuse may not be seen as being as harmful as physical abuse, it is, in fact, just as devastating, and the person committing it is just as dangerous. Attacking a person's self-esteem is the most common form of psychological abuse. This can take the shape of attacking a person's looks, calling them fat, ugly, skinny, or any other derogatory term that makes them feel inferior to others. It can also take the shape of attacking a person's abilities, such as their intellect, memory, or ability to perform certain tasks.

Low Self-Esteem Behavior

Codependent behaviors can also come from the side of the victim of a codependent relationship. In these cases, the behaviors are not abusive; instead, they are subservient in both form and purpose. After all, codependency is a two-way street, requiring both a taker and a giver. Therefore, it is just as common for givers to practice codependent behaviors in all of their relationships as it is for takers to do the same. Although the behaviors practiced by givers are safer and even more beneficial in appearance, they are nonetheless just as dysfunctional. They need to be fixed just as much as the behaviors demonstrated by takers.

More often than not, the behaviors demonstrated by givers come in the form of low self-esteem behaviors. One such example is the need to please other people. Again, this behavior unto itself is not necessarily a bad thing. After all, any good friend will want to make sure their friends are happy and cared for. However, it is the extreme nature of the behavior that points to codependency. Wanting to please people from time to time is fine, but needing to please everybody all of the time is something else altogether. Yet, this is the nature of codependent behavior, as demonstrated by givers. Any time you see someone endlessly trying to please everyone around them, you know, they are a giver, so they need help. The very same thing applies if you find yourself feeling the need to always please everyone around you all of the time.

This behavior can be taken to the next level in more extreme cases where the giver feels the need not just to please everyone, but to fix the problems in everyone else's lives. The compulsive need to fix other people's problems is a classic sign of codependent behavior on the giver. Again, any good friend will want to offer advice when someone is having issues in life; however, a codependent person will not only provide advice; they will want to step in and save the day. This need to fix other people's lives is dangerous, as it not only creates undue stress on the giver, but it also creates undue stress on those whose lives they are trying to fix. More often than not, the giver will try to step in and take charge, feeling as though their efforts are normal, and the outcome will justify the means. This can result in them being overbearing, something that can mask the identity of a giver as givers are usually subservient and passive.

Denial Behavior

The third type of codependent behavior is what is known as denial behaviors. This is where the individual cannot accept the reality of a situation, and thus rewrites reality to suit their needs. Such behavior can be demonstrated by both the giver and taker in a codependent relationship. The main difference between the two is that the taker rewrites reality to make themselves look better. In contrast, the giver rewrites reality to make others look better. In either case, the core behavior is denying what is real and replacing it with something that the individual finds more desirable.

Perhaps the most common of denial behaviors is that of denial itself. In the case of the taker, this comes in the form of denying their responsibility anytime something goes wrong. Even when all the facts are blatantly obvious and point to the taker being solely responsible for a situation, they will deny that they are to blame in any way, shape, or form. This denial can often be seen when a taker loses their job. Even if they are fired for poor performance, breaking policy, or some other reason that is their fault alone, they will deny the facts and blame something else altogether. They may choose to blame the economy, stating that their company was downsizing but chose to fire them to avoid paying unemployment. Even worse, they may accept that their performance was to blame, but they will blame their home life for their poor performance, thus shifting blame to someone else, such as a spouse or parent. In any event, they will never allow blame to fall squarely on their shoulders. Instead, they will deny their role in anything that goes wrong, no matter how obvious that role may be.

Finally, there is the denial behavior of unrealistic hopes. When a person denies realistic hopes and expectations, choosing instead to believe in something completely based on fantasy and imagination. In the case of the taker, this behavior takes the form of the belief that all the things that are wrong in life will somehow resolve themselves without any effort on the part of the individual. Thus, rather than taking responsibility for their role in events, the taker will rely on a savior riding in and rescuing them from a life beneath their true worth. Alternatively, a giver will live in the delusion that their situation will improve when the takers in their life realize the error of their ways and begin to live normal, healthy lives. Unfortunately, this is never likely to happen, yet rather than accepting the inevitability of their situation, givers will hold out hope for the proverbial miracle that will rescue them from their life of suffering.

Victim Behavior

The final type of codependent behavior to consider is what is referred to as victim behavior. This is where the individual, both taker and giver alike, view themselves as the victim in the relationship and act accordingly. In both cases, this behavior is intended to engender sympathy and support, providing the individual with the boost they need to feel better about themselves. However, victim behavior only ever enables both parties to be at their worst, thereby perpetuating a codependent relationship in which all parties suffer.

In the case of the taker, one of the most common types of victim behavior practiced is hypochondria. This has its roots in hospital settings where victims of injury or disease became addicted to the care and support provided by those around them and thus chose to be in a constant state of pain or sickness to continue receiving that care and support. However, hypochondriac behavior extends into every environment, including work, home, and anywhere that a codependent relationship can exist. The bottom line is that the taker will create some issue that justifies their inability to care for themselves, while also creating the need to be cared for by another. It can come in the form of actual physical illness or suffering, or it can come in the form of a general inability to be self-sufficient. Ignorance, fear of failure, insecurity, and the like can be used as an excuse to shirk responsibilities and acquire extra care and attention from the giver. In short, a taker will use anything to create sympathy, which is what they crave most of all.

Finally, there is the victim behavior known as a martyr mentality. This behavior can be practiced by both takers and givers alike. In the case of the taker, the individual creates a narrative in which they sacrifice everything for the happiness and wellbeing of others. Ironically, this is them projecting the actual role of the giver onto themselves. Even more ironic, the giver usually feeds into this narrative, thanking the taker for their sacrifices, even though such sacrifices usually do not have any basis in reality. For example, a taker may claim that by marrying their giver-spouse, they gave up many other dreams that they would have pursued otherwise.

CHAPTER 3 - Types of Codependent Relationships

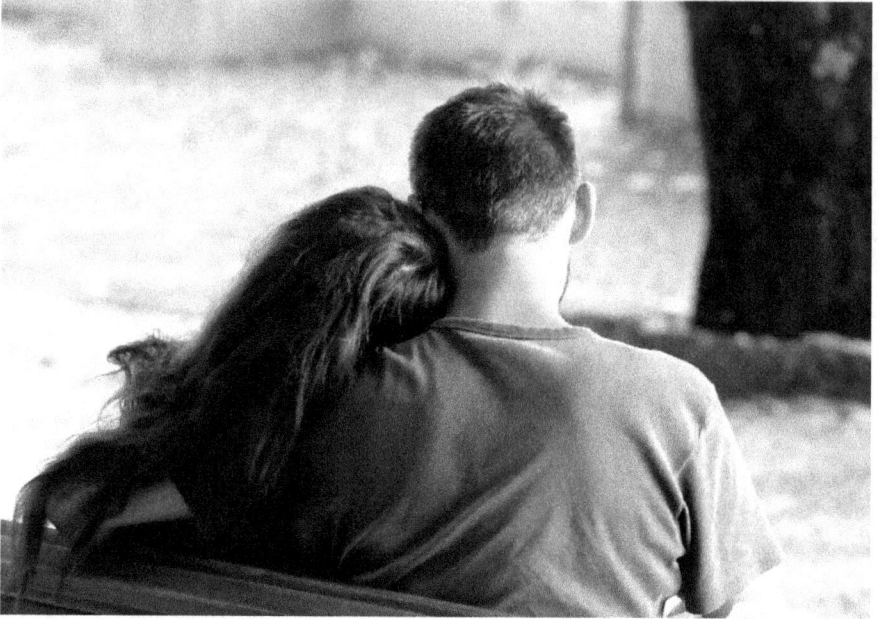

If you are in a relationship that is not healthy, do not get down on yourself. Studies show that as much as 80% of relationships are dysfunctional to some extent. If you are in a healthy relationship,
you are likely in the minority. Relationships act as a mirror to ourselves. If we are unable to be in a healthy relationship with ourselves, if we are able to love ourselves and then, this will only be exasperated by our intimate relationships with others.

The dysfunction and codependent patterns that we have inherited from our parents and created to cope with childhood trauma are magnified and expressed in our intimate relationships.

Being in a relationship that is intimate can be scary and can reveal all of our deepest insecurities, but a healthy relationship can give you the support and inspiration to become your truest self.

Three Types of Codependent Relationships

Typically, codependent relationships tend to fall into three categories—the rescuer, the supporter, or the confidante. These categories describe the different ways in which a person falls into familiar roles when interacting with another person who brings out their codependent conditioning. A person who struggles with addiction or dysfunctional behavior brings out the codependent tendencies in their partner. One person takes on the giver-rescuer role, while the other undertakes the taker-victim position.

The Rescuer

The rescuer is the person who derives their sense of self and worth by attempting to rescue or save others. They will continually attract themselves to people and situations in which they feel compelled to make tremendous sacrifices to help others. Unfortunately, these people who they compulsively attempt to save are often individuals who are themselves attracted to partners who will enable them. Both the rescuer and the rescued depend on each other and require each other to continue their compulsive and addictive behavior.

The Supporter

The supporter is similar to the rescuer; the difference is that they do not try to rescue the person who is filling the taker wrong; instead, they support the other person in there addictive or dysfunctional behavior. Another word for this is enabler—this person supports and enables the other rather than having strong personal boundaries and being honest with the other person. Often, they do this because, from a young age, they were forced into a role of supporting a dysfunctional parent, and so this is how they have learned how to express their love and be loved in return.

The Confidante

The confidante is one who listens and empathizes with a dysfunctional or addicted partner. While it is helpful and compassionate to listen to another and be there for them, it is not helpful to validate another's incorrect and unhealthy behavior. The confidante attends a level of feeling needed and valued by the fact that they are there to commiserate with their addicted partner.

The Codependency Trap

The fact is that codependent individuals are attracted to other codependent individuals. When two people with the same illness are brought together into a relationship, there is no chance for a healthy union, which allows both individuals to grow and heal.

Signs of a Codependent Relationship

Common signs of codependency in a relationship are:

- Chaotic and intense interpersonal relationships

- A fear of being alone which manifests as attempts to continually be in a relationship

- Persistent feelings of emptiness and boredom

- Allowing one's own needs to be secondary to the person youare in a relationship with

- Intense and out of balance need for affection and acceptance

- The ceaseless need for perfection

- Always needing to check with someone or something outsideof oneself before making choices

- Chronic dishonesty and denial of what is going on

- Patterns of manipulation

- Lack of trust in the relationship

- One or both patterns exhibiting a low self-worth.

What Is a Healthy Relationship?

The great poet Kahlil Gibran said that to people in an intimate relationship must be like two pillars of a temple, who together hold up the roof but do not stand too close to each other or else they will interfere with each other's life journey. Like two trees, they must have their own space so that their routes do not fight over the soil's nutrients. A healthy relationship supports you and being your best self, but it does not exist to make you happy or to live your life for you.

People often enter into relationships not as equal individuals who can share intimacy without dependence and needing something from the other, but as wounded and insecure people who are seeking someone outside of them to fill a gap and a hole that they feel inside. A codependent individual's dysfunction is expressed in their relationships, and it is through the building of healthy relationships that you finally free yourself from negative beliefs and patterns of dysfunction.

Being a Healthy Individual

To have a healthy relationship and have a healthy and fulfilling life, you must become a whole individual. People who have developed codependent habits due to their childhood experiences do not learn how to be autonomous, independent individuals.

A psychologist called this process of being your true, authentic self—individuation. A person who has undergone individuation has defined themselves as a unique individual who is not dependent upon their parents or any other person outside of themselves. They are following their unique path in life and have a healthy sense of self. Many times, people criticize the ego, but the truth is you must have a developed and strong ego to live in this world and not become controlled and made into a victim by others. Codependence does not have this strong and defined ego and, as a result, mold themselves like a chameleon to whatever they believe others want them to be. Individuation is very important for healthy relationships because the greater you are an autonomous individual, the more you can experience true intimacy with your partner. Contrary to what some believe, true intimacy is not being the same in the dissolution of all boundaries but is the result of two whole individuals coming together in equality. Additionally, people are happier in their relationships to the degree they have developed their self-identity and self-esteem. Finally, people are drawn to partners who are at an equal level of individuation as the elves, so if you are codependent, you will attract a codependent mate. However, if you are a healthy, autonomous adult, you will naturally find yourselfmaking partnerships with others who are equally mature and healthy.

Intimacy and Autonomy

It is a common trait of codependent relationships that there is no healthy amount of both intimacy and autonomy. The two go together.To be truly intimate, there must be two individuals. Codependent individuals commonly think of themselves in relationships as either "you" or "we," and they completely lose sight of their "I." Since theydo not have a strong sense of self and ability to be happy on their own,they come to attempt to find a sense of wholeness through union withthe other person.

These people will give up their whole life to spend every moment with their partner. They will start seeing their friends and sees engaging inhobbies and interests. They expect their partner likewise to drop all outside activities and interests to spend all their time together. If theirpartner wishes to spend some time independently, hanging out with friends, they will be hurt and may make the other partner feel guilty for wishing to spend time alone. Most times, this results in a lack of respect and not honoring boundaries and the other person's need for time for themselves and their other relationships. This causes resentment in the partner as they feel that they are being controlled and that their partner wishes to change them.

The same phenomena can be seen in reverse. In this case, one of the partners feels threatened by intimacy, and so they try to emphasize their identity and individuality while pushing their partner away. They are hypersensitive to being controlled and do not have a strong sense of identity either. This just goes to show that someone can be codependent and exhibit the opposite end of the spectrum. On one side, someone tears unworthy of love and so pushes their partner away. On the other side, someone feels terrified of aloneness and so desperately clings to their relationship.

At the root of all these struggles with autonomy and intimacy is the individual sense of self and how they feel worthy of being loved. It is an interesting character that the more you are capable of being alone, the more you are capable of being in a relationship. The more you are autonomous, the deeper you can go into intimacy.

Relationships with this imbalanced state often turn into power struggles about everything, whether it be chores, work, relatives, or friends. It is very common for relationships to be stuck in this conflict pattern for many years until finally, one partner cannot take it anymore and leaves.

What Makes for a Healthy Relationship?

The unfortunate truth is that many people who struggle with codependency are not able to accurately evaluate a partner to see if they are healthy and someone that they can enter into a functional relationship with.

Due to their early life experiences, they associate dysfunctional behavior as normal and perhaps even feel safe and comfortable being in a relationship with someone who is unhealthy just because that is familiar to them.

The following are some traits of healthy and long-lasting relationships. Of course, not all couples can fill all of these requirements all the time.

However, a healthy relationship should follow these guidelines the vast majority of the time.

- Both partners feel safe

- Both partners make decisions together

- Both continually develop their Self and their self-esteem

- Realistic expectations

- Effective communication

- Acceptance of the other's differences and needs

- A balance of quality time together and alone

- Cooperation and mutual giving

- Both partners maintain outside friendships

- The sharing of a common vision for the relationship

- Have similar values and needs.

CHAPTER 4 - Detaching From Codependent Influences

The number one rule of breaking free from a codependent relationship recognizes that you can never change the other person. Only when you come to terms with this fact can you
begin to take the measures necessary to liberate yourself from the influences and effects of a dysfunctional relationship. One such measure is to practice what is referred to as detachment. Simply put, detachment is the process of removing yourself from the codependent equation. This can be achieved by avoiding arguments, ending the role of being responsible for other peoples' happiness, or by stopping any other action that contributes to the codependent nature of the relationship.

Recognize You Aren't Responsible for Other Peoples'

Happiness

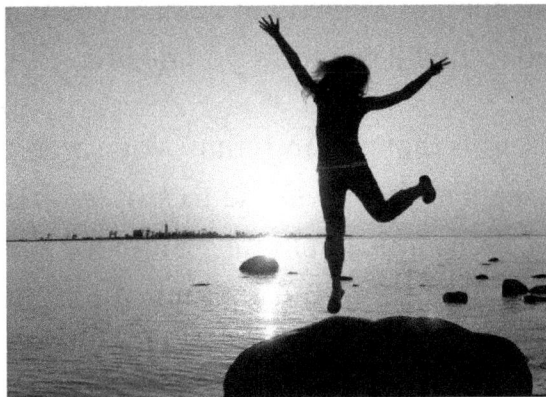

Questa foto di Autore sconosciuto è concesso in

The first step toward achieving detachment is to change your way of thinking. This covers a wide range of areas, so it cannot be done all at once. Instead, it is a process that must be achieved one step at a time. While there is no wrong place to start as such, perhaps the easiest and most important place to start changing your way of thinking is regarding other people's happiness. The bottom line is that you aren't responsible for how other people feel, no matter what others might say. Only when you realize can you begin to move on with your life in a healthy and meaningful way.

This change in mindset will take a while to develop, as your current mindset is probably the result of years of conditioning. Subsequently, you mustn't look for immediate results. Instead, treat this the way you would if you were trying to develop muscle strength or lose weight.

You wouldn't expect to walk into the gym one or two times and come out looking like a bodybuilder. Similarly, you wouldn't expect to eat a salad or two and miraculously drop ten or twenty pounds of extra weight. Instead, you recognize that any meaningful results will take time. Therefore, expect these results to take the same time and effort. This way, you can commit to the long game, allowing yourself the time needed to make progress you desire.

The easiest way to begin recognizing that you aren't responsible for other peoples' happiness is to stop taking responsibility for all of their choices simply. Suppose the taker in your relationship relies on you making the right decisions to be happy and start demanding that they begin to share in the decision-making process. This doesn't have to bean all or nothing scenario; rather, it can be a step by step process in which you slowly turn over the burden of responsibility to the other person for finding happiness in their life. You might start by forcing them to choose between a few options rather than making all the choices yourself. For example, if you plan to go out on a date, instead of making every decision yourself, come up with a few options you think might work and make the other person choose one. This is a perfect balance that allows both parties to make decisions together, rather than relying on one person to be fully in charge.

Recognize You Aren't Responsible for Other Peoples' Unhappiness

The next step toward detaching from codependent influences isrecognizing that you aren't responsible for other peoples' unhappiness. Again, this is all about realizing that every person is ultimately responsible for how they feel, both happy and otherwise. Unfortunately, in the case of a codependent relationship, you will be made to take the blame for when the taker is unhappy, no matter whatthe reason might be. Even if you aren't directly responsible for the action or situation that causes their unhappiness, the taker will still blame you for not protecting them more effectively from those thingsthat brought them misery. This is about as unrealistic a mindset as you could imagine, one that usually creates a sense of hopelessness on thepart of the giver. After all, you can't possibly protect a person from everything that might cause them to become unhappy, no matter howhard you try. Therefore, the mission is as impossible as it is hopeless.

To put this overwhelming hopelessness behind you once and for all, you need to begin to change your perspective on things. Again, you must understand that no individual is responsible for someone clsc'shappiness, sadness, or any other state of mind. Therefore, do not feedinto the narrative that you are to blame when the taker in the relationship is angry, sad, or depressed. Instead, take a step back andrecognize the impact that the taker's choices had on their overall emotional wellbeing. The chances are you can trace their unhappiness to their past choices or behavior. Once you do this, you realize that their unhappiness results from their own actions, not yours. After a while, you will start to see a pattern, one that reveals the simple truththat the taker is solely responsible for their overall wellbeing. This will help you to change your perspective on things, thereby freeing you from the guilt for failing to protect others from being unhappy. The bottom line is that you didn't fail; therefore, you are guilt-free.

Begin to Make Decisions for Yourself

The basic lesson to be learned concerning how a person feels is that it all comes down to the decisions the individual makes. When a person makes good, positive choices, then they are likely to be happy and content with their life. Alternatively, when they make bad, negative choices, they will be unhappy and frustrated with their day-to-day existence. That said, now that you have freed yourself from the idea that you are responsible for how other people feel, the next step toward detachment from codependent influences is to start making decisions for yourself. This not only allows you to break free from the cycle of codependency, but it also enables you to move forward with your life, creating a life of happiness, fulfillment, and meaning. By making decisions for yourself, you can start to shape your life in a way you never imagined possible!

You might find this process difficult to get used to at first. This is because you have probably spent most of your life feeling as though every decision you made had to be about everyone else and not about you. The chances are you never took the time to consider how you felt about the choices you had to make. Instead, you looked at the options you had to choose from and tried to decide which option would be more pleasing to the other people in your life. In a way, it's a bit like constantly Christmas shopping for other people. Every decision you made was an attempt to bring happiness to others and never bring happiness to yourself.

To move on with your life, you need to begin to turn that thought process around and start making decisions for yourself rather than for other people. Only then can you truly be free of the controlling influences of a codependent relationship?

Become Self-Aware

As a result, you may find it difficult to choose yourself since you may not know what things you like and what things you do not like.

The idea of becoming self-aware might sound like some Zen ideal that requires hours of meditation or yoga to achieve. Fortunately, while meditation and yoga can help to achieve a deep level of self- awareness, they aren't required for the level you need at this point. Rather than needing to find out your place in the Universe, the self-awareness you are looking for right now is what your favorite color, or what ice cream flavor you like the most. As such, the path to this level of self-awareness can be a fun and exciting one, requiring more daring than discipline, as in meditation or yoga! The trick is to treat this as a time of self-discovery, one that allows you to meet yourself for the very first time.

Since most choices are subjective in nature, there isn't a right or wrong answer. Instead, it comes down to a matter of preference. This is especially true in the case of what your favorite color is or what your favorite ice cream is. At first, you might feel anxious when trying to make decisions on such matters as you probably do not know the answers. However, rather than stressing out about it, simply explore life, making one choice at a time, and learning as much as you can along the way. For example, do not be afraid to try different flavors and colors until you find the ones that work for you. The choices you make in life should bring you joy; therefore, find the things that make you happy and then start choosing them regularly. If you choose that isn't happy, do not feel as though you failed or made a mistake. Instead, recognize that choice isn't right for you and do not make it again.

Accept the Truth

The most important lesson to learn is that the other person in your relationship is probably beyond changing; thus, any time and effort you spend trying to fix them will prove wasted. In fact, the more you try to fix the taker in a codependent relationship, the worse things will usually get. Takers do not want to heal; they only want to keep taking. This goes back to the example of the sick person never recovering in a hospital. Such a person doesn't want to get healthy since getting healthy means having to take care of themselves and losing the support of the giver. Therefore, they want to stay sick so that they can be cared for continually. Trying to fix them is ignoring the fundamental truth that they want to remain broken.

Furthermore, trying to fix other people is one of the main behaviors of a giver, making it a codependent tendency. If you want to detach from codependent influences, you must eliminate any behaviors within your own life that would enable a codependent relationship, including the urge to fix other people. Therefore, rather than trying to fix the relationship and everyone involved, the key is to fix yourself, thereby removing yourself from the equation and thus ending the cycle of codependency. Only by accepting this truth can you effectively let go of the codependent influences in your life and begin to move on, creating a life of freedom and happiness for yourself.

CHAPTER 5 - Establishing Independence

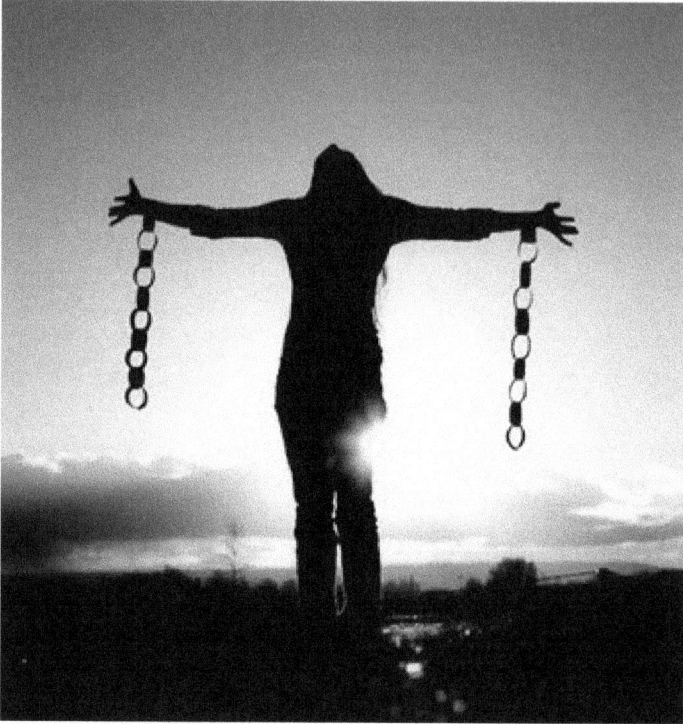

Aperson may choose to end a life of codependency for a number of reasons. However, even though these reasons may differ in appearance, they usually boil down to two main goals.

The first goal is to escape the abuse that comes from a codependent relationship. The need to be free from abuse of any kind is often enough to motivate a person to free themselves from any codependent relationships they find themselves in. The second goal that inspires a person to escape codependency is to establish independence. When a person is trapped in a codependent relationship, they spend their lives serving others' needs and desires. Once they decide they want to spend their lives pursuing their personal goals and ambitions, it becomes necessary to escape any codependent relationships. Only then can the individual be free from the burden of serving others and begin to live a life for themselves, one that enables them to pursue their dreams and find the happiness they deserve.

Define Yourself as an Individual

The next step is to take the items that made the cut, namely those that belong to you and create a new list. This new list will be the start of your new life, one that is focused on chasing those dreams that come from your heart and mind, not the heart and mind of another person. You may find a very small number of items on this list, which shouldn't concern you. The real aim of this exercise isn't to discover your dreams; rather, it is to differentiate them from those dreams that do not belong to you. Once you make this distinction, you can clear your heart and mind of the ambitions that came from others, thereby making room for those hopes and desires that are yours and yours alone. This will enable you to focus your energies on those things that will bring happiness and meaning into your life, thus creating the life you deserve.

Discover Your Hopes and Dreams

After you have cleared your mind of the thoughts, hopes, desires, and dreams that weren't yours, you can begin to fill it with those that truly do belong to you. However, most people at this stage struggle to come up with a list of any significance, both in terms of length and substance. The few items they can list out usually seem fairly trivial, especially compared to the grandiose schemes they had been expected to fulfill on behalf of the taker in their codependent relationships. This is perfectly normal, as anyone who has been in a codependent relationship will have turned their mind off to anything that was self-serving and focused their attention and efforts instead of things that served the taker in the relationship. More often than not, the average giver doesn't have the time or the motivation to contemplate personal goals. Therefore, they find that their mind is blank when they go to write out any personal goals or dreams once they achieve their freedom codependency. Therefore, at this point, you need to take the time to discover those things that you want to do now that your life is yours once again. The first step to discovering your hopes and dreams is to sit down and ask yourself one simple question, "If I could do anything with my life, what would I do?" Some people struggle to find any answers at all to this question at first. Again, this is particularly true for anyone who has spent a great deal of time as a giver in a codependent relationship. In this case, the trick is to give yourself the time you need to find the answers. It may come down to spending time in the outside world to find inspiration and ideas. After all, most victims of codependent relationships live very sheltered and controlled lives. Therefore, they do not always know the options that are available to them when it comes to creating an independent life. The important thing is to take all the time you need to find what inspires you. Once you find inspiration, be sure to write it down so that you can start pursuing that goal and finding the happiness that you deserve.

Alternatively, some people find that they have many ideas and dreams to put down on their list. The problem most of these people face is that many of those ideas and dreams seem unrealistic, as though they are the product of an overly active imagination. This may, in fact, be true to a large degree since many victims of codependent relationships create a vivid fantasy world in which they can escape the pain and suffering they experience in their real life. It can be all too tempting not to write down such dreams and ideas, dismissing them as too unrealistic or ridiculous to admit, let alone consider pursuing. However, it is vital that you write down every idea and dream you have, no matter how fantastic or unrealistic it may be. The objective here isn't to create your life plan; instead, it is simple to discover your innermost hopes and desires. Therefore, write down any and every dream you have, even if it is to become king or queen of the world!

Determine Your Direction

Now that you have compiled a list of your hopes and dreams, you can begin to take the next step to determine your direction. Depending on what your dreams and goals are, you might only need to consider getting a better job or a better place to live.

The important thing here isn't to create a goal simply for the sake of
creating a goal. Instead, it is to create a goal that will bring the most happiness and meaning into your life. This is why it is important to create a clear list of all of your hopes and dreams. This list will present certain patterns, and it is those patterns that will determine the direction you need to take to achieve the life of your dreams. For some people, the list will consist largely of things oriented around a job or career. Whether it's about making more money, finding a more challenging job, or pursuing the career of your dreams, in this case, your direction will be job-oriented. This means that you need to spend your time and efforts pursuing everything you need to get that dream job, including training, education, and even contacts who might help you to get your foot in the proverbial door.

Alternatively, your list might consist of items of a different nature, such as making friends, finding a person to share your life with, or even starting a family. If your list pattern is more about love and friendship than of money and career, you need to steer your life in the appropriate direction. Rather than spending all of your time fixated on your job or your finances, you need to spend your time and efforts socializing. Start spending time with any friends you currently have, especially in such settings like parties or social gatherings where you can meet new people. By exposing yourself to more people, you can start to make new friends or even start looking to engage in relationships of a more intimate nature. The key is to break out of the bubble you lived in as a victim of codependency and begin to expand your social and romantic horizons. If love and friendship are where you will find happiness, then you need to make those your new priorities in life.

Create a Plan

Once you have determined the direction your life needs to take to become a happy and fulfilling life, you both desire and deserve, the next and final step to achieving independence is to create a plan. While determining a direction and creating a plan may seem to be the same,they are two distinctly different processes. The process of determining direction allows you to develop the overall goal that will bring happiness into your life. This is a general idea as it was. In contrast, creating a plan is the process of laying out a step-by-step approach that will enable you to achieve your goal.

A good analogy of this is the planning of a vacation. When you plan a vacation, the first thing you do is decide the type of vacation you want. You might want to spend a week hiking in the woods, skiing in the mountains, or just lounging around on a beach. Deciding the type of vacation you want is the same thing as determining the direction in your life. The next step is to choose a specific destination and plan on how you will get there. You might need to book a flight if your destination is a long way off. If your destination is closer to the home,you might only need to choose the route you will drive to get to whereyou want to be. This is the process of creating a plan.

If getting a better job is all that it will take to make your life a happy and content one, the plan would be to look around at all available jobs. If any of them jump out at you, then you move to the next phase, namely filling out any necessary applications or other paperwork and pursuing an interview. The important thing is to focus all of your time and energy on achieving your goal, being sure to take each of the necessary steps carefully and thoughtfully, thereby giving yourself the best chance of success. Researching the best methods for creating resumes or taking interviews, for example, might be another step you take to increase your chances of success.

Finally, suppose you are the type of person who requires something greater than a regular job or the happiness that friends or a family can provide. In that case, you will need to create a more intricate and lengthy plan, one that will launch you from the shallows of your codependent past into the stratosphere of your ultimate dreams. Such a plan will doubtlessly involve the pursuit of higher education. Even before you start applying to colleges and universities, the first thing you will probably need to do is determine the finances you need for such an education. The next step will be to look for scholarships, grants, and loans that will provide the funds you need to for your higher education. After all, there is no point in applying to a college if you can't afford to go.

CHAPTER 6 - Establishing Healthy Relationships

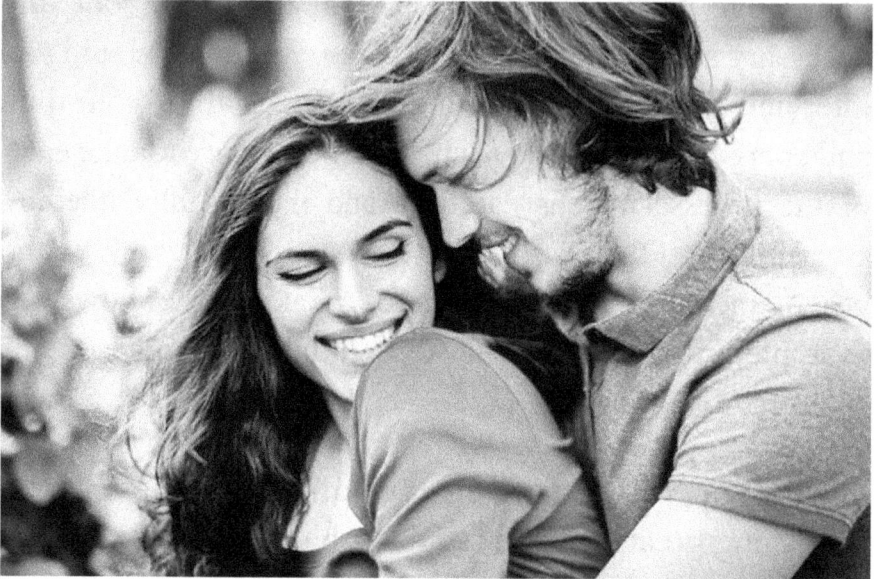

Now that you're able to define the line where your partner ends and where you begin, you can now open yourself to the idea of mending the relationship or entering a new relationship as
a more confident, more assertive person.

- How to deal with the dependent spouse during recovery

- How to deal with friends and family during recovery

- How to begin a new relationship while recovering.

The Dependent Spouse

Now that you're on your way towards recovery, your partner will naturally begin to notice the difference in you. You will hear complaints like "You've changed." or "You've become selfish." A dependent spouse may blame it on your therapist or on the 12-step program that you're taking. When this happens, respond to the confrontation with: "Yes, I have changed. I'm taking better care of myself, and there's nothing wrong with that." Remember to meet your partner with calm assertiveness. Eventually, your spouse's challenging behavior will pass.

If your partner is an addict, keep in mind that mending the relationship can't be possible unless he is also on his way to recovery. If you're getting help, then he should too, and so should everyone else in the family who is affected. During this time, remember that the addict's addiction problems belong to him and him alone. Thus, do not waste your energy and time trying to solve it. Instead, use them to focus on yourself, your kids, your career, or your passions.

Once your spouse reaches a stage of sobriety, there will be a "honeymoon phase." However, all the anger, guilt, and fears of the past will always be lurking in the shadows. It is important to note that you should NOT bring up the past to your recovering partner. There's no point in reminding them of their mistakes when they were under the influence of the addictive substance. You'll accomplish nothing apart from shaming them and undermining their progress.

Another issue that codependents usually face when the addicted spouse is starting to recover is relinquishing their dominant position in the household. As the dependent begins taking in more responsibilities in the marriage, you may find it hard to let go of the power. Allow your partner to stand on his/her own two feet and take pride in knowing that he/she can once again contribute to the relationship or the family.

As you begin to learn who you are as a person, you can form your likes and dislikes. You are more aware of your wants and needs. This may mean that you have to re-introduce yourself to your partner. Talk about your similarities and your differences and learn to respect them. Take pride in the fact that you are no longer just mirroring your partner's personality. You can be yourself—no apologies needed. Adjustments have to be made to honor the differences in both your preferences. Give each other plenty of affection. But give each other plenty of space as well.

In the bedroom, codependents usually assume the role of the pleaser or the giver. You may find it difficult just to relax and become the receiver. You are afraid of becoming vulnerable. You are afraid of not being in control. As a result, you end up performing sex as though it were a chore. Your spouse will feel this, and he/she will lose/ or has already lost interest in engaging in sexual relations with you. Healthy sex in a marriage or a relationship requires not just physical intimacy but also emotional and spiritual closeness. Talk to your lover about intimacy in the bedroom. Discuss the things that you like and the things that you do not like. Make a list of things that you would both like to explore. This way, sex doesn't end up being one-sided. Instead, it becomes a physically, emotionally, and spiritually satisfying act that can strengthen your relationship.

Letting Go

When you establish boundaries, anticipate that people are going to test them. When you find that the relationship (whether it's with your spouse/your friend/your parents, etc.) is no longer working and that the person keeps making attempts to violate your boundaries, then it's time to move on.

Consider that as a codependent, you have lived in misery. And as the saying goes: "Misery loves company." But what happens when you're no longer miserable? You will naturally seek out a company that is happier, more assertive, and more supportive. As you change, so do your needs. This includes your social needs. You may need to sever ties with your abusive lover, family, or a friend or spend less time with them. Sometimes, achieving full recovery requires cutting yourself off from the past and moving in an entirely new circle so that you can avoid persons and relationships that can undermine your progress or cause you to relapse.

Dating

Qualities to look for in a potential partner:

- Honest

- Reliable and trustworthy

- Respectful

- Open

- Has the ability to establish clear boundaries

- A good listener

- Supportive

- Genuine
- Caring

- Understanding

- Knows how to compromise

- Independent (can care for himself/herself)

- Has healthy social connections (friends/family).

You may be wondering: Do I deserve such a person? Yes! You do.

Now that you know that you deserve better, it's only natural to want to be in a healthy and equal intimate relationship. You're becoming healthier, and so you are looking for prospective partners who are as healthy as you. It's okay. You have so much love to give, and you can't keep it bottled inside you forever. More than that, dating while recovering can do wonders for your self-esteem.

However, here's a cliché though very effective advice: Take it slow. If you have sex with a casual acquaintance, it would be wrong to form expectations around your sexual partner. Unrealistic and, therefore, unmet expectations will only lead to disappointment and a feeling like you have been used. This can cause you to regress to your old habits. What to do? Find out first if it's possible for you to develop a friendship.

Refrain from having sex when you feel…

- Threatened

- Afraid

- Obligated

- Manipulated.

Likewise, avoid using sex to win a person's love or to manipulate
someone.

When your body is telling you to stop, then do not be afraid to verbalize it. Say, "Stop." Say, "No." If you notice that you're trying to justify your sexual behavior, then stop doing it. Remember that it is only you and you alone who possess the right to decide who, when, and whether or not someone may touch you.

Ingredients for Sustaining a Healthy Relationship:

- A healthy dose of self-esteem

- Effective and assertive communication

- Realistic expectations

- Respect and acceptance

- Mutual decision-making and problem-solving

- Cooperation

- Time together and time apart

- Compatible values

- Common long-term goals.

CHAPTER 7 - How to Salvage a Codependent Relationship

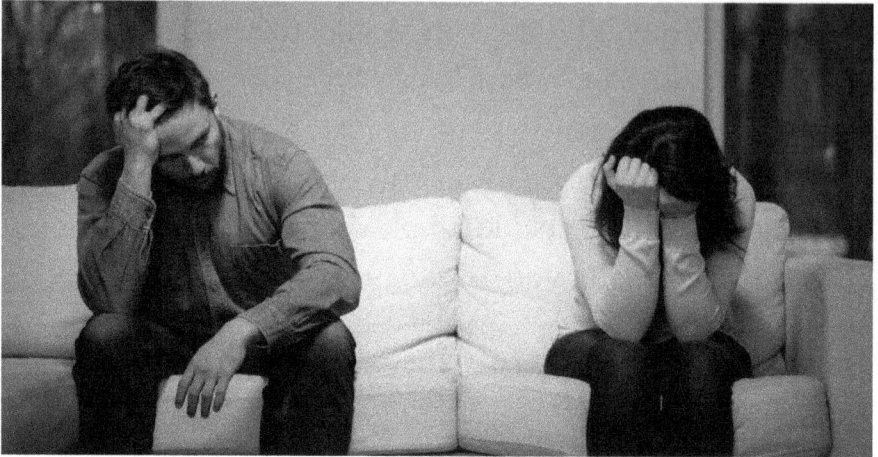

Acodependent affair may be extraordinarily deplorable for thecodependent individual and rest around that individual. The individual on whom you are codependent probably will not

have a ton to recognize after the nonattendance of care or desire to not comprehend particular of the grant components of codependency. A codependent individual will begin disregarding their prosperity, set wrong needs for the duration of regular day-to-day existence, and relentlessly make rancor everlasting and for everything around that individual.

The Best Technique to Correct Codependent Ties Initiates With Recognizing Codependency

1.   You ought to recognize codependency and recognize thatyou are codependent. This is tough just as someone is dependent on a different person, either truly or rationally, fiscally, or in a greater number of ways than one. But if an individual recognizes that the individual being referred to is codependent, one won't have the will or the arrangement to fix the issue.

2.   When codependency is recognized, a line or a couple of lines be going to be strained. All codependent conduct must stop. In this case, if a life partner has an alcoholic spouse, then the wife should not like the husband paying little heed to how crushed he is. This may be burdensometo do anyway; it must be affected. A line must be drawn.If a man has a narcissist sister, by then, he ought to stop driving the narcissistic conduct. As opposed to pushing orsubbing for the narcissist sister's conduct, the kin shouldempower her to recognize the cold hard truth of the world. In a wide scope of codependency, the codependent individual accomplishes various objects, which are not tothe best bit of leeway of the relationship and, without a doubt, not strong to the codependent person. Each should not engage codependency by footing the offender,dependent individual, or one with a character issue. As opposed to engaging, every single encouraging movement or feedback should be ended instantly.

3.   A result must be chosen. That may not be careful toward the began anyway by and significantly a month or months, one must choose to see the completion of the entry. Do you intend to linger in the relationship? Do you the inclination to leave the relationship and establish another life? Do you wish to recover the relationship? The reaction to these requests would choose how uncommon or how evaluated a procedure you should have.

4.   Searching for master aids is significant for all things considered. Codependent people are likely not going to be adequately ready to catch up alone. Months or significant lots of codependency make by far remarkably powerless- willed and besides engrave the confidence. Searching for or having capable aids will implement a codependent individual to have an aching and the self-restraint to see by way of catastrophes.

5.   Huge than anything, one needs to fix the purpose behind codependency. The secret of mending a codependent rapport distorting in the patching could be substance abuse, mental issues, or character issue. The essential driver has disposed of, never again insist codependency continue, nor would the glue is a codependent relationship. Revamping the rule issue is significantly more troublesome than one may anticipate. It requires some investment to discard alcoholism or a long time and a huge amount of attempt and master aid to fix

character or mental issues. Regardless, this is likewise the terrific means to deal with amend a codependent relationship. There is simply unusually a great deal of an individual can supposedly and request to manage to locate the issues of codependency if the fundamental concern actuating codependency continues.

6.   It may not work by and large work, yet conversing with the individual with whom one offers a codependent relationship may be a tricky concept. In case the other individual is adjusted or efficient and if the relationship is commonly fulfilling in various habits, then discussing and having a collective procedure can be very helpful. A concerted means is compelling since both the people in the relationship would then have the option to make some little walks, in their specific habits conferring to their scope and quality, to patch the issue. Right when two people cooperate, it has a huge mental influence, which is altogether constructive. Conversing with an alcoholic life partner, sitting and watching out for the issues, persuading someone to forgo substance exploit, or if an individual recognizes their blunder of physically misusing the other individual and after that stops it, by then how to mend a codependent relationship turns into a cakewalk.

7.   Fixing a codependent relationship necessitates a long trip. It is a long walk around the circumstance. Additionally, that walk is not basic. Having a belief is indispensable, and one should, in like manner, be completely conscious of the charming conclusion. There is nothing incorrectly with removing a codependent relationship, as it is definitely common to patch it. It is imperative to have a conventional, genuinely strong system as watchmen, companions, family relatives, or someone who can give the quality and continue rousing one to continue further,conquer every trouble.

How Might I Quit Being Codependent in a Relationship?

Enable Consequences to Happen

If your accomplice is late for work since he's been pulled over for a DUI, do not delude the boss for him. Allow the trademark consequences of his moves to take place. Once in a while, the primary way an addict can give indications of progress is by hitting "outright base," and that can't happen if someone is continually covering for them.

Guidelines to Stop Being an Engaging Codependent Operator: Know Your Cutoff Points

Comprehend that "NO." is a complete sentence. Recognize what your cutoff focuses are and stick to them. One way to deal with do this is to channel your body for your one of a kind notions. Acknowledge when something makes you uncomfortable and give yourself the approval to put a stop to it, paying little respect to whether it might make your accomplice upset. Make sense of how to offer need to your special slants of comfort, instead of constantly endeavoring to fulfill your accomplice.

Stop Being Codependent: Focus on Yourself

This is a significant one. Become increasingly familiar with yourself better. Discover what you like and what you do not and find out how to fill your reality with a more prominent measure of what you like. Make courses of action with companions, and do not hold up until you understand your accomplice is difficult to reach to make plans! Guarantee that you are practicing self-care (eating extraordinary, working out, getting enough rest, etc.) and empowering time to discover relaxation exercises that you welcome that exclude your accomplice.

Connect

Understanding that you aren't in this situation alone is an incredibly astonishing resource. It can help you with feeling less isolated, and it might even empower you to recognize other individuals who accomplish fundamentally the same as things that you do. This will empower you to become conscious of why you think and feel that way that you do. It's very retouching to recognize why you act the way you do; this is what we call "becoming conscious," and it's the pathway to enthusiastic chance.

Look to Your Past

The underlying advance on your approach to security is to research your one of a kind past to uncover and comprehend encounters that may have contributed to your codependency. What is your family heritage? Is there eager negligence and abuse? Were there events that provoked you isolating yourself from your genuine internal emotionsand ignoring your very own needs?

This can be a problematic strategy and one that incorporates contemplating and re-encountering youth sentiments. You may even find that you feel angry, awful, terrible, or accountable as you consider this.

Recognize Renouncing

The second way to repairing is to genuinely be straightforward with yourself and recognize the issue. There doubtlessly a phenomenal plausibility you have intellectualized and upheld your codependence after some time. While it can feel alarming to confess to being codependent and connected with a messed-up relationship, dependability to yourself is very the underlying push toward patching.

Disengage and Disentangle Yourself

To truly wear down and create ourselves, we have to at a first disconnect from the things we are messed with. Personal development will require giving up our interruption and over-consideration with endeavoring to control, rescue, or change others and our defaulting to continually endeavoring to fulfill someone else.

This infers taking a full breath, surrendering, and recognizing we can't fix that is not so much our own to fix. What issues do we "have" and what issues are "asserted" by others in our lives? It's about genuinely endeavoring to isolate where you end and others start.

Practice Self-care

Self-care means managing ourselves physically—eating healthy, getting enough rest, rehearsing ordinarily, and taking off to our PCP and taking any recommended drugs. Self-care in like manner means contemplating ourselves deep down, making social connections, discovering happy, positive activities to fill our time, and allowing ourselves energetic get-away and lay in case we need it. It is like manner suggests connecting and taking a gander at our very own considerations, sentiments, characteristics, needs, and needs—paying little regard to what other's conclusions are. Extraordinary systems to do this can be composing and reflecting through journaling, examining appropriate reference on self-care, and of course, going to treatment. To make a strong whole deal relationship with others, you should first create a strong one with yourself.

Make Sense of How-to Express No!

Presumably, the best ways you can begin to characterize sound limits is to make sense of how to object to conditions that are hurting to your one of a kind thriving. This will feel uncomfortable from the beginning, yet the more you do it, the less complex it will become. We save the benefit to oppose others, and normally, we do not need to give them a long explanation. We hold the choice to object to things that are not the best for us. This isn't connected to being intolerant and barbarous towards others—yet it's connected as far as possible and putting our one of a kind needs first.

Be Self-Caring First

Be minding to yourself! This is about self-compassion and treating yourself a comparable way you would treat the others you appreciate!

You ought to be big-hearted to yourself consequently. Treat yourself as you would treat a companion who is persevering. Make sense of how to challenge any negative, essential self-talk and any negative convictions about yourself and your confidence.

Learn Independence

Finally, go at secluding from others for explicit periods to make a sound sentiment of self-rule. Decrease dependence through making sense of how to be removed from every other person and truly making sense of how to like it! Codependent people consistently believe that it is hard to contribute vitality alone without others around them.

CHAPTER 8 - How Can Codependency Ruin Relationships?

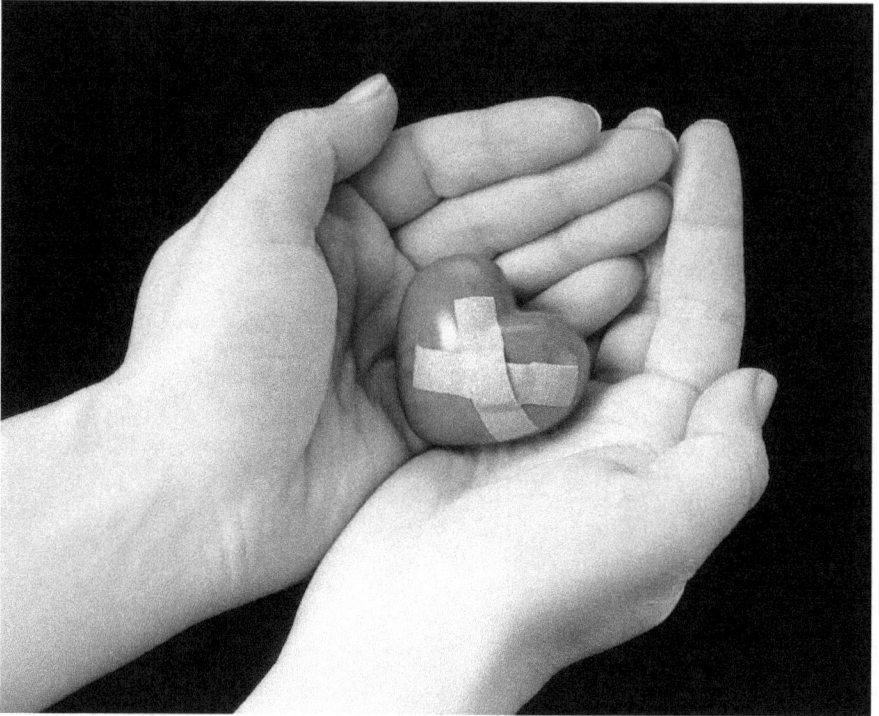

Codependents lack a healthy sense of self. They are ultimately lost within themselves. They are prone to put others first rather than have their own needs fulfilled. Codependents are the
people who have trouble accessing their internal cues, and so they think and behave differently around another person.

This includes people who are addicts, or processes such as sex addiction, gambling, or substance abuse such as food disorders or any other kind of addiction. The need to use or consume starts with the feeling of emptiness and damage done in childhood, often concealed by a sense of devalued self, shame, emotional abandonment. Children adapt to the environment in different ways to survive, and one of the ways to soothe yourself is to adapt to other people.

In this case, their thinking and behavior begin to revolve around another person, similar to how some teenagers might turn towards substance or video addiction. It used to be music. Now it's gaming, internet, and phones. They use it to soothe themselves because of the pain, anxiety, depression, or whatever is going on internally.

The Development of a Codependent

This is the same way, and for many of the same reasons, someone who is codependent turns toward another individual. When a child is raised by parents who lack empathy and mutuality, they will try to make themselves visible to the adults and attempt to find out what will keep them safe. They discover whether they need to achieve or please, depending on the child's personality.

The more the codependent goes through these changes to survive their emotional selves, whether in the form of using drugs or adapting to someone else, the larger the gap becomes between their real self and codependent self. They eventually develop a default zone. It can be a leader, a rebel, hero of the family, or any such role that they may develop. That becomes their personality. Maybe they are always trying to tell jokes, whether to distract their parents from fighting or make them laugh. The more the person does this, the farther they get from their real selves. Authenticity becomes a distant memory.

This has much to do with their levels of neglect or punishment when they were growing up. Even well-meaning parents, who may not have been overtly abusive, can sometimes use shame tactics with their children by being intense. Similar to physical violence—sexual abuse can also play a role.

There is a phenomenon called the trauma of images of invisibility. Children will ask the adult about their childhood and think it was fine. They remember going on vacations, and that they had everything they needed. They went to good schools, but their parents existed in an emotional vacuum. In this case, avoid develops, and children do not get the closeness and emotional attachment they need to thrive. They learn to not turn to their parents for comfort, or even when they are feeling distressed.

These parents are often well-meaning; they are too busy with each other, work, financial stress, or any other reasons they may have. But their actions, even unintentional, can cause a child to start to feel ashamed of their feelings, which are very integral to who we are as a human being. To become a whole individual, we form an identity with our thoughts and feelings, perceptions, and beliefs. We can become an asset—distinguishing us from what our parents want and their beliefs in their raising of us.

This is called the individuating. We become separate. If parents are depressed and codependent, they may even raise their children to become codependents. Because their parents aren't emotionally available, they are unable to meet their needs.

Shame doesn't come into play as an emotional concept until you are over a year old. There are different studies where some say that it isn't until after a child three years old, where may show disgust or their bowel movements may change. These are signs.

Babies are forming their relationships and emotions, but most people do not think of babies as individuals. They are, and they form their identity concerning someone else, just like therapy is a process based on the reaction from another person to heal our identity in a relationship with somebody else. People have a lot of cognitive distortions. Because perceptions are usually formed by what we are taught or what we experience, the result often comes from faulty parenting.

When a parent is raging at a child, they believe that they are a terrible child. Maybe parents aren't even saying anything; they are just busy on their phones. This can cause the child to become emotionally distant. It is necessary to tell your children and help them believe that they matter to their parents. They need to feel and understand that each parent wants a relationship with them, and not just because they are performing well in school or they are soccer stars, but for who they authentically are.

Children shouldn't be turned away from when they are crying, or think that they are bad because their parents are angry. Parents need to make them feel that they are accepted and that their parents honestly want to spend time with them. It is only by a demonstration that a parent creates a child's interest in values. It's good to have it coming from one parent, but still, it's not enough, because it creates trauma in his mind when he doesn't have it from both of his parents.

Sometimes when one sibling gets more attention than the other, the one left out may start to feel more like an outsider in the family. This can also happen when the parents are fair, but their siblings are narcissistic. They may be teasing them, abusing them, or even physically hurting them, and parents are at fault for not intervening and not protecting them. This again makes the child think that there'ssomething wrong with them.

Enter Codependency

Codependency can be thought of as a secondary condition. It's a symptom of deeper problems. When we evaluate codependency, it isnot the problem itself that we treat, but rather a problem caused by something much deeper. Therapists are better equipped to work to solve the problem. Codependency is a product of not only a deep shame but more along the lines as a response to trauma. The type of trauma is called attachment trauma. It occurs during the early years ofone's life when they are bonding with their parents.

Children of narcissistic parents observe and do what makes their parents happy, and ultimately get some semblance of what they want.But what they do not get is the feeling of self-worth. They start to experience a sense of deep loneliness. They develop a relationship template that is about giving to others to feel love or comfort in one's skin. That relationship template is then taken and is manifested into codependency. At the very core of a codependent is the sense of loneliness. It is deeply painful. It burns with pain. The only way thatthe codependent can often find love is with a narcissist. They find thatthis style of relationship takes away the loneliness and makes them feel comfortable. The codependent feels complete.

In reality, this is a relationship comprised of two underdeveloped people. It can be referred to as a half-person relationship because they need each other to feel good and feel whole. That's why their relationship starts up so quickly, intensely, and often sexually. To feel complete and whole in the world in which they live, they need to connect to another person.

Talk to any codependent, and they will tell you that outside of a relationship, the feeling of intense loneliness becomes something that cannot help but be focused upon. This loneliness can often be traced back to attachment trauma. But the codependent avoids the loneliness by becoming attracted to the narcissist. Even though it is dysfunctional, the loneliness is held at bay. When they are facing a situation of leaving the narcissist, the narcissist leaves them, or they should be alone, they fall back into feeling lonely. This loneliness is their number one withdrawal symptom. Codependency is like an addiction because a codependent needs a relationship with a narcissist to feel real euphoria. They feel like they have a place on this Earth. They belong to someone even though that person is troubled.

CHAPTER 9 - Factors That Sustain Codependency

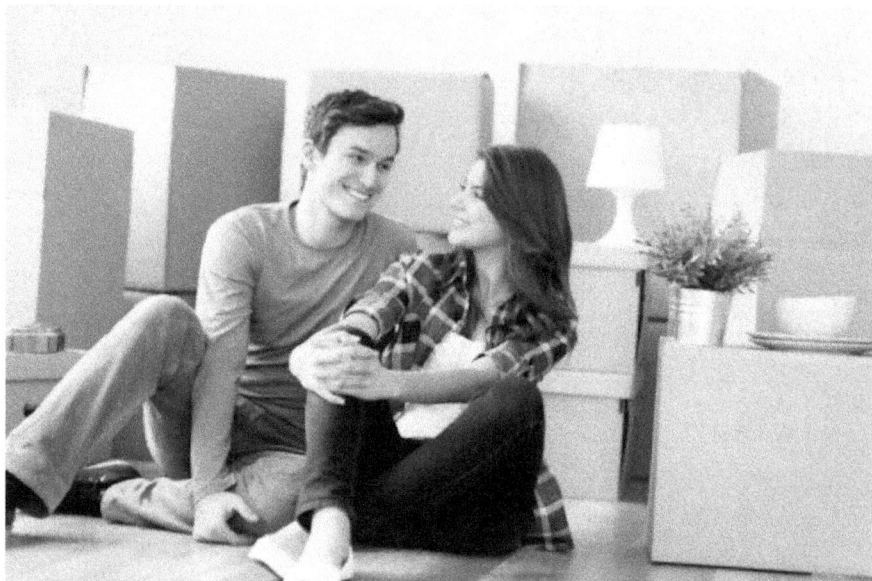

Often codependency continues to perpetuate due to different reasons. As a codependent person, you must make an effort to understand the reasons that sustain codependency so that

you can look for ways to overcome those. You are your enemy, and which is why you struggle to overcome codependency. Sabotaging yourself becomes a constant thing assuming that you do not deserve a good life. Of course, you might have made some mistakes in your past; who doesn't? But not forgiving yourself for past mistakes is not the right decision. You start denying your strengths and thoughts. There are different ways of self-sabotage, including codependency, aggression, abusive relationships, denial, and more.

Even after realizing codependency, you will not be able to overcome it because of self-sabotage, which can make you feel unworthy, which triggers codependency even deeper. To treat codependency, you must believe that you are worthy. You should think of the way a person with self-love would handle the situation that you are in. A person with self-love will not select unhealthy options that might hurt their mind and body.

If you can't love yourself yet, try to fake it for some time, and so you will gradually make it true. Self-sabotaging is closing the actual view, which is why you are struggling to see the reality, so when you fake it, you will be able to clear the path slowly, but firmly. If you consider factors like anger, denial, and shame, they perpetuate codependency pretty easily. Hence, you must educate yourself about the factors so you can overcome them.

Anger and Denial Regarding Codependency and Your Partner

Denial Your Partner's Behavior

Denying your partner's behavior is one of the common denials, but you can overcome it. You deny that your partner is addicted, and his or her addiction causes many problems in your life. Yet, you are not ready to accept it, which is why codependency perpetuates in your life. This kind of denial is common because codependents have been facing similar situations from their childhood. They might have grown up with parents who are addicts, so it looks normal to them.

The addicts and dependents have gotten used to been taken care of, so they are not ready to take responsibility. And codependents are okay with that because they like to take care of others.

If you deny your partner's behaviors, you must understand that you are walking towards a dangerous destination. You must acknowledge the reality and work accordingly because a relationship can ruin your life if you do not handle it wisely. You must accept the fact that you are not responsible for their behaviors. If they are addicted or relying on you for almost everything, it means you have created the path for it. You should not let anyone hurt you just because you are codependent. If you deny your partner's behaviors, it doesn't mean that you do not care about them. Of course, you are bothered, but you just do not see the seriousness, or you somehow build up reasons to justify the act. This is the typical behavior of someone who loves their partner, but the love codependents show extra. They do not make an effort to correct the mistakes; they just ignore them. However, ignorance will make things worse.

Denial of Codependency

When you are confronted about codependency, you will deny it, and that's the very first step. You can see that you are codependent, but you are not ready to accept it because you think it's a situation that has made you a codependent. You try to blame the situation and people so that you do not have to discuss codependency. Most codependents do not want to discuss it because they think it will worsen the pain, but it will not. This is one of the reasons why you deny that you are codependent.

Another reason is you are not someone who seeks help from others, so if you accept that you are codependent, you'd have to get help from others to treat it. This kind of mentality leads you towards a destructive path. You do not like the fact that someone is taking care of you and being responsible for your behaviors because, for a long time, you've been doing it for others. You do not want others to make you happy as it triggers self-examination at a point. When you are codependent, you can easily avoid self-examination, which is why you turned down help from others.

Denying your true nature, which is codependency, will help you to stay away from professional help and admitting your codependent nature. On the other hand, some codependents do not seek professional help, but they try to treat themselves all alone. They believe that they can find out the problem by talking to close friends and reading reliable books and articles. But sometimes, this can be dangerous depending on the level of codependency that you have. You may be ashamed to seek help, so you try not to get in touch with professionals. But remember, it is not a wise move.

Denial of Feelings

This is another type of denial which deals with a codependent's feelings. You are not ready to discuss how you feel, and ultimately, you end up denying your feelings. Normally, codependents can easily understand what other people feel and worry about. Plus, codependents spend a lot of time helping others to feel better. But they deny their feelings, which create resentment in their hearts. Codependency gives rise to obsession. When you are obsessed, you get distracted from what's important. Similarly, when you are obsessed with your partner, it will be hard to focus on your feelings because you are worried about your partner's feelings more than yours. If you think about your feelings and how you have been doing, you will have no solid answers because you have denied your feelings. Even if you understand your physical pain, you will not understand emotional pain because you are blinded by codependency. Growing up, you have not had an environment that lets you share your emotions and feelings. You may have always been the one to listen, not the one to speak. Moreover, you do not understand why you should share your feelings when nobody is there to comfort or listen. Hence you keep denying your feelings from childhood. Feelings serve a purpose even if they are not positive feelings. Through feelings, you understand what you need and do not. If you want to interact with people, you must have the ability to share your feelings.

How do feelings help you become better at interacting while overcoming codependency?

- If you are angry, you will be reacting to make changes.

- If you are sad, you will empathize and value human connections.

- If you fear, you will keep dangers at bay even if they are emotional dangers.

- If you are guilty, you will have values that you respect.

- If you feel ashamed, you will not harm others.

- If you feel lonely, you will strengthen your connection with others.

Likewise, every negative feeling serves a purpose. When you deny your feelings, you won't be able to move forward in life. You will bottle up your feelings for years, and it will always be there in your subconscious mind. When you accumulate pain, you will not be able to overcome it. Instead, constant denial might be your answer. What will happen when you continue to deny your feelings? You will end up depressed, and depression isn't as easy as you think!

Maybe you do not, but most codependents treat resentment as a shield to hide anger. Of course, your past or childhood would have been unpleasant and difficult. Maybe you couldn't express what you feel because nobody bothered to listen, but that doesn't mean it will repeat in the future unless you want it to repeat. If you stop denying your feelings, you will be able to lead a healthy and happy life. It is important to talk to your partner and explain how you feel because, unlike other healthy relationships, your partner will not understand your feelings. Not because he or she doesn't understand others, but because you have been hiding your feelings from them.

Unresolved feelings will repeat itself. If you overcome denial and anger, you will be able to overcome codependency too. But if you do not, it will perpetuate. And you must learn about the snowball effect to understand sustaining codependency.

The Snowball Effect

We all have dealt with the snowball effect in life. Many times in life, you would have dealt with situations that you thought wouldn't blow up this big, but before you know it, the situation becomes a huge mess. This is symbolic of a snowball that rolls down the hill and forms something huge. Just like that, the negative feelings and thoughts about yourself can snowball into something huge, and before you know it, there would have been a huge mess. You will not be able to cope with yourself when the snowball gets

93

smashed and creates a huge mess! Certain thoughts make the whole process of opening up to yourpartner difficult, and some of them are:

• You tend to jump to conclusions without focusing on theevidence.

• You tend to generalize even if you see a single negativething to support certain activities.

• You often catastrophize because you only think about theworst possible outcome.

• You easily filter the positive things into negative.

• You set strict rules regarding the unrealistic expectation ofyours and others.

These negative feelings will increase your anxiety and enhance your negative mindset. When your mind is filtered through these feelings, it can be complicated to see things in the right way. You will not makean effort to change or to motivate yourself to overcome codependency because your mind is filtered that way. If negative emotions and behaviors snowball down the hill, you will not stop it successfully. Hence, you must stop it when it started. Well, stopping the snowballwhere it started might impossible, but it is not. If you follow a few essential points, you will be able to do it.

- The critical point is to break the chain. Start by challenging a few thoughts and looking at them objectively.

- Write your feelings down or talk to a close friend about it. Also, when talking to them about your feelings, if they have something to say, let them because listening is also essential.

- Do not skip your day-to-day activities because when you have a routine, you will distract negative thinking for sometime.

- Engage in mindful activities, exercises, and yoga.

These tips might look simple, but they are not as easy as they sound because consistency and patience are two essential things when you are trying to overcome codependency. If you try to move out of this vicious cycle in one go, you are likely to get hurt. Instead, baby steps will help you overcome codependency without creating a mess. Do not let your mind snowball in the process of healing, so even the process of healing should be done step by step.

CONCLUSION

Compromise is an important part of a relationship.

What you should always do is have an open and honest dialogue. On the other hand, we also show you that compromise doesn't mean you lose your voice and lose who you are. We emphasize that you should be able to be who you are in your relationship and that you shouldn't get lost. We help you understand how you can keep yourself in your relationship by making sure you don't get lost. We also teach you and give you helpful tips and advice on why you should accept your partner for who they are and why it's important to make sure you appreciate them for who they are.

Good luck.

CPSIA information can be obtained
at www.ICGtesting.com
Printed in the USA
BVHW090333040521
606332BV00006B/1067

9 781801 869744